Epsom Salt

Tremendous Benefits & Proven Recipes for Your Health, Beauty and Home

www.amazon.com/author/kira-novac

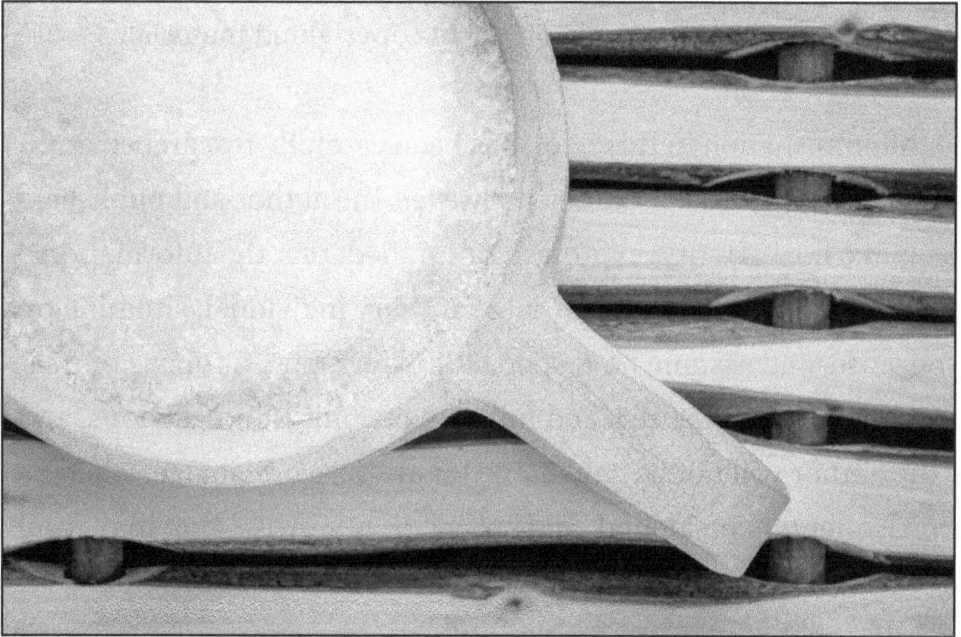

All information in this book has been carefully researched and checked for factual accuracy. However, the author and publishers make no warranty, expressed or implied, that the information contained herein is appropriate for every individual, situation or purpose, and assume no responsibility for errors or omission. The reader assumes the risk and full responsibility for all actions, and the author will not be held liable for any loss or damage, whether consequential, incidental, and special or otherwise, that may result from the information presented in this publication.

A physician has not written the information in this book. Before making any serious dietary changes, I advise you to consult with your physician first.

Free Complimentary Recipe eBook

Thank you so much for taking an interest in my work!

As a thank you, I would love to offer you a free complimentary recipe eBook to help you achieve vibrant health. It will teach you how to prepare amazingly tasty and healthy gluten-free treats so that you never feel deprived or bored again!

As a special bonus, you will be able to receive all my future books (kindle format) for free or only $0.99.

Download your free recipe eBook here:

http://bit.ly/gluten-free-desserts-book

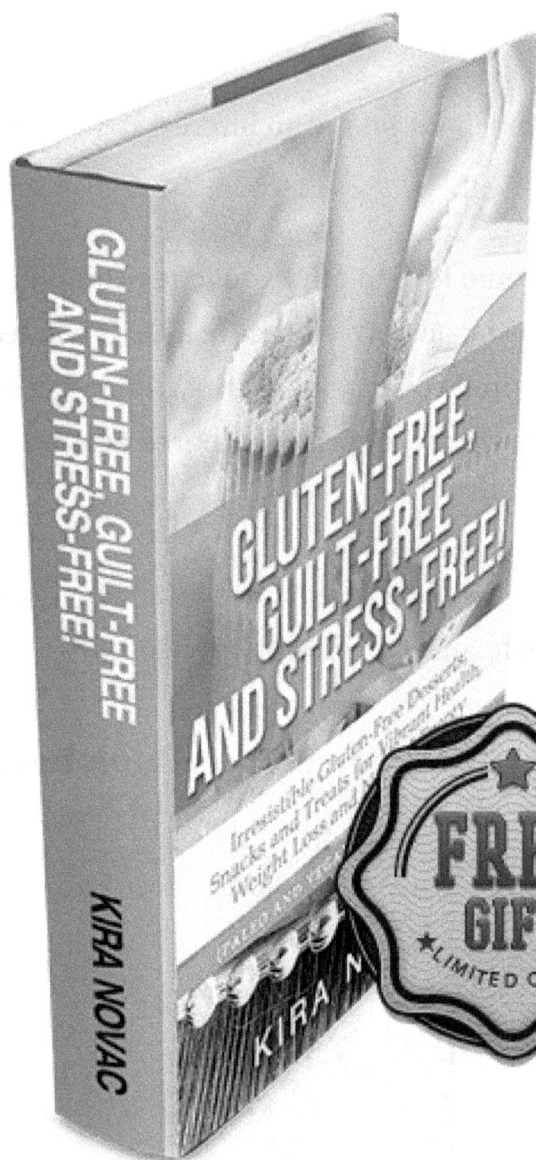

GLUTEN-FREE, GUILT-FREE AND STRESS-FREE!

GLUTEN-FREE, GUILT-FREE AND STRESS-FREE!

Irresistible Gluten-Free Desserts, Snacks and Treats for Vibrant Health, Weight Loss and Vitality

KIRA NOVAC

KIRA N

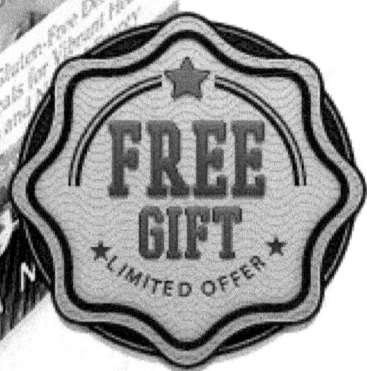

FREE GIFT

LIMITED OFFER

Table of contents

Introduction

Epsom salt, which gets its name from the bitter saline spring in Surrey, England, it is not actually a salt as such but rather a mineral compound that is naturally occurring and is a compound of magnesium and sulfate. Epsom salt has a myriad of benefits and can be used in the treatment of ailments, in beauty routines, around the house and in the garden.

There are extensive studies that have shown how magnesium and sulfate is readily absorbed by the body through its biggest organ, the skin. Which is why an Epsom salt bath is the easiest way to enjoy the many health benefits of this mineral combination; magnesium is an essential mineral that plays a role in so many different activities that naturally occur within the body. These activities include the reduction of inflammation, aiding muscle and nerve function, and the prevention of the hardening of arteries. Sulfates help improve the absorption of nutrients, ease headaches and migraines, as well as flush out toxins from the body's entire system.

Epsom salt is also known for its ability to help relieve pain and cramping, regulate blood sugar, remove splinters, relieve sprains and bruises, relieve constipation, and relieve the symptoms and discomfort of gout. It can also be used to treat toenail fungus and athlete's foot.

Epsom salt is also known for its many uses within a beauty regime, which include exfoliating the skin, naturally cleansing the skin and removing blackheads, removing the buildup of styling products and adding volume to your hair, as well as removing foot odor.

Around the house Epsom salt can be used to clean pots and pans, clean tiles and grouting, and remove the buildup of cleaning products and detergent in your washing machine, as well as being used as a hand wash. Epsom salt can be used in the garden as a natural fertilizer and for the prevention of slugs. It is also a natural and organic means of preventing insect infestations within your garden.

Epsom salt is an affordable, natural way of treating, preventing and aiding so many different essential daily activities and the chapters to follow will show you many easy and creative ways to use this gift of nature in just about all of your everyday activities and necessities.

This book is divided into four chapters that will cover the different uses of Epsom salt as well as provide you with recipes on how to put together useful combinations using Epsom salt as your base. These four chapters will cover the use of Epsom salt for health, beauty, home and garden and their combined use with essential oils.

Chapter One: Epsom Salt for Your Health

Epsom Salt has so many uses when it comes to everyday health ailments. This chapter will show how you can use this natural, affordable ingredient to treat and prevent some of life's everyday health concerns and incidents.

One of the most effective ways to reap the benefits of Epsom salts for your health is to include an Epsom salt bath two to three times a week in your normal routine. For a relaxing, stress relieving bath do the following:

1. Draw a warm or hot bath to the temperature that you most desire, but make sure the water isn't too cold
2. Add 2 cups (500ml) of Epsom salt to the bath
3. Using your hand, swirl the Epsom salt around in the water in order to make sure that all has dissolved into the water
4. Soak in the bath for at least twelve minutes

Epsom Salt for Arthritic Joints and Gout

An Epsom salt bath is a wonderful way to ease the symptoms of arthritic joints, this is due to its high magnesium content; magnesium is an essential mineral that is known for its ability to help regulate fluid and acid retention within the joints and therefore ease swelling, both symptoms of arthritis. To use Epsom salt for the relief of painful arthritic joints do the following:

1. Draw a warm or hot bath to the temperature that you most desire, but make sure the water isn't too cold or too hot
2. Add 2 cups (500ml) of Epsom salt to the bath
3. Using your hand, swirl the Epsom salt around in the water in order to make sure that all has dissolved into the water
4. Soak in the bath for at least twelve minutes
5. While in the bath, move your joints around in the warm water as much as possible in order to get the blood flowing within your joints and muscle tissue
6. After moving your joints around for approximately five minutes, begin to gently massage your joints and muscle tissue while keeping the area that you are massaging under water
7. Once you have finished with your Epsom salt bath, dry off and try to relax for at least two hours in order to allow your

joints and muscle tissue to reap the benefits of the Epsom salt bath as well as the massaging that you gave them.

8. This kind of bath is best taken just before bed.

Epsom Salt for Athlete's Foot

Epsom salt also has a use for its antifungal properties and therefore can be used as a natural remedy for the treatment and prevention of athlete's foot, which is a fungal infection that commonly attacks the skin on the underside of the feet and can also cause a fungal infection within the bed of the toenail. Eucalyptus oil is an essential oil that is native to Australia and is known for its anti-bacterial properties, by combining it with Epsom salt to treat fungal infections such as athlete's foot; you are creating a natural and soothing treatment for this ailment. To use Epsom salt for the treatment of athlete's foot do the following:

1. Fill a plastic basin, or the bottom of the bath with warm water (deep enough to submerge both your feet up to ankle height)
2. Add 1 Cup (250ml) of Epsom Salt
3. Add approximately 10-15 drops of Eucalyptus oil
4. Soak your feet in this solution for approximately 15 minutes
5. Dry off your feet, making sure that they are completely dry as fungal infections such as this thrive in warm and damp environments
6. It would be best to allow yourself time to put your feet up for about one hour after this, allowing them to breath (so you should remain barefoot) and relax

Epsom Salt to Help Relive Constipation

Epsom salt has become known for its use as a saline laxative, which is a natural and non-evasive way of treating constipation. Many laxative treatments can be rather hard on the body and the more chemical based ones tend to cause the long term side-effect of the body becoming reliant on a chemical laxative in order for natural bowel movement to take place. Using Epsom salt to remedy constipation won't have this side effect and will work by simply adding a little more lubrication to the peristaltic movement of the bowel, which is the process by which the bowel and colon naturally breaks down food in order to move it through the intestine and discard of waste products; when you are constipated this natural process is not occurring efficiently and therefore may need a little help. To use Epsom salt as a remedy for constipation do the following:

1. Dissolve 1 teaspoon (5ml) of Epsom salt into 1 Cup (125ml) of warm water
2. Drink
3. It is important to note that this remedy should not be used more than once per day and would be best done either first thing in the morning or just before bed time

4. If this remedy does not relieve your constipation within three days, then it is recommended that you consult with your doctor.

Epsom Salt to Soothe Sprains and Bruises

Sprains and bruises are everyday occurrences and can happen without us even trying too hard; simply stepping off the bus at the wrong angle could cause a minor sprain or twist in your ankle, and a simple bump of the knee against your desk drawer could cause a bruise. Of course there are also the more serious sprains and bruises that can be a result of injuries caused during sporting activities, minor accidents and general household activities. Epsom salt provides a natural remedy for such ailments by doing the following:

1. Draw a warm or hot bath to the temperature that you most desire, but make sure the water isn't too cold or too hot
2. Add 2 cups (500ml) of Epsom salt to the bath
3. Using your hand, swirl the Epsom salt around in the water in order to make sure that all has dissolved into the water
4. Soak in the bath for at least twelve minutes
5. Once you have finished with your Epsom salt bath, dry off and try to relax for at least two hours in order to allow your sprains and bruises to reap the benefits of the combination of the warm water and Epsom salt
6. This kind of bath is best taken just before bed.

Epsom Salt for Arterial Health

It is widely thought that Epsom salt has the ability to prevent serious cardiovascular illnesses by decreasing inflammation and protecting the elasticity of the arteries. Healthier arteries mean that there is less risk of plaque build-up within the arteries or damage to the arterial walls. One of the most common causes of many health ailments that are heart related is the highly stressful lives that we lead. Stress and emotional fatigue affects the body in so many ways and can be just as silent a killer as high cholesterol or diabetes, this is why it is so important to take time out to relax and invigorate the body; after all we only have one body and if we don't take care of it, it can't take care of us. Regularly soaking in a warm bath with Epsom salts can help relieve and reduce stress, therefore helping to relieve the many health problems that come with excessive amounts of stress. In order to use Epsom salts as a supplement to arterial health and the reduction of stress do the following at least three times per week:

1. Draw a warm or hot bath to the temperature that you most desire, but make sure the water isn't too cold or too hot
2. Add 2 cups (500ml) of Epsom salt to the bath
3. Using your hand, swirl the Epsom salt around in the water in order to make sure that all has dissolved into the water
4. Soak in the bath for at least twelve minutes

5. Once you have finished with your Epsom salt bath, dry off and try to relax for at least two hours in order to allow your body to reap the benefits of your relaxing bath.

6. Try to keep warm and still

7. This kind of bath is best taken just before bed.

Epsom Salt to help Remove Splinters:

Splinters are another everyday occurrence that can sometimes be very difficult to prevent or side-step. As simple an act as grabbing the broomstick to sweep the kitchen floor could leave you with a splinter in your finger; hanging the laundry with wooden clothes pegs could also cause this. Most of the time a splinter will be close to the surface of the skin and therefore easy to dislodge, but sometimes it can go deeper, making it painful and hard to remove. Epsom salt can help in this case by performing the following:

1. Dissolve 1 teaspoon (5ml) of Epsom salt into 1 Cup (250ml) of warm water

2. Soak the splinter containing body part in the warm water/Epsom salt solution for about 5 minutes

3. The magnesium sulfate in the Epsom salt will reduce the inflammation around the splinter as well as softening the skin and the splinter, making it easier to remove

4. Using a regular sewing needle that you have disinfected by placing in boiling water, carefully remove the splinter by sliding the sharp end of the needle underneath the skin and underneath the splinter

5. Once you have the needle underneath the splinter it should be easy to just slip it out of the skin.

6. Rinse the affected area off with clean water and place a plaster or band aid over it if necessary

Chapter Two: Epsom Salt for Beauty

Epsom salt is an affordable and natural ingredient that will benefit any beauty routine and it is well worth considering doing so. This chapter will give you some ideas and recipes for natural, non-evasive beauty routines that use Epsom salt as their base.

Epsom Salt for moisturizing the skin

One of the most common beauty concerns is achieving an adequate moisture balance of the skin. The moisture levels of our skin can be affected by a number of factors including ageing and the change in season. When our skin loses moisture, it also tends to lose elasticity, which can cause premature ageing. There are also other skin ailments that can result in dry, itchy skin such as eczema or psoriasis. When combining Epsom salt with a non-evasive or natural moisturizing ingredient you are able to treat dry skin and its symptoms without causing further discomfort or irritation. Very often moisturizing creams and lotions contain high levels of fragrances and chemical additives, which can be very irritating to sensitive skin, often making the problem worse. Here is a natural remedy using Epsom salt and extra virgin coconut oil to moisturize the skin. Coconut oil is not only known for its heart healthy fat content when using it in cooking and baking, but it is also known for its beauty benefits and is a natural way of effectively moisturizing your skin. To use the combination of Epsom salt and coconut oil to moisturize your skin do the following:

1. Draw a warm or hot bath to the temperature that you most desire, but make sure the water isn't too cold or too hot
2. Add 2 cups (500ml) of Epsom salt to the bath
3. Add ½ Cup (125ml) of extra virgin coconut oil
4. Using your hand, swirl the Epsom salt around in the water in order to make sure that all has dissolved into the water, and that the coconut oil is evenly distributed
5. Soak in the bath for at least twelve minutes
6. Once you have finished with your Epsom salt bath, pat your skin dry as rubbing with the towel can cause irritation to the skin.
7. Dress warmly, covering as much of your skin as possible in order to allow it to further absorb the coconut oil
8. This kind of bath is best taken just before bed.

Epsom Salt for exfoliating the skin:

Regular exfoliation of the skin is necessary in order to rid it of dry and dead skin cells that may be sitting on the surface layer. By exfoliating the skin, we are not only ensuring that it is cleansed properly, but also ensuring that it is able to adequately absorb any moisturizing products that we are using. Regular exfoliating of the skin also helps it to look healthier and prevents it from becoming dull and lackluster. Many commercial exfoliating products have a tendency to be very harsh on the skin and in many cases they may over exfoliate the skin causing redness, inflammation and further drying out of the skin.

For those who suffer from sensitive skin, commercial exfoliating products can be very evasive and cause incredible discomfort and further sensitivity, also the high fragrance content of many of these products can not only add to skin sensitivity but can also cause the skin to dry out even more. Epsom salt provides you with a natural, non-evasive and gentle way of exfoliating your skin allowing you to gently remove excess dead skin cells without overdoing it. Exfoliating of the whole body is best done in the shower when the skin is damp and then followed by the use of a moisturizer. To naturally and non-evasively exfoliate your skin and then effectively moisturize it afterward, do the following.

1. Take 1 Cup (250ml) of Epsom Salt

2. Get in the shower and dampen your skin

3. Grab a handful of Epsom salt and gently rub it over your skin using your hands

4. Rinse off all the Epsom salt, taking care to make sure that you have removed all the salt from your skin

5. Finish your shower routine as usual

6. Once you are finished in the shower, pat off excess water using a damp face cloth

7. Before you get out of the shower, rub some extra virgin coconut oil over your body

8. Pat your skin dry with your towel and dress warmly making sure that as much of your skin is covered in order to lock in the moisture you have given it from the coconut oil, which will be effectively absorbed due to the exfoliating you had done prior to rubbing on the oil

9. It's best to do this routine just before bed time since our skin naturally repairs itself while we are sleeping and therefore it will be able to fully reap the benefits of the beauty routine that you have just performed.

10. If you experience any skin discomfort, it may be that you were too harsh with the rubbing of the Epsom salt on your skin, so next time try being a little gentler. However, if you do find further discomfort after trying this routine a second time, then it is possible that your skin is too sensitive to

exfoliation as some people do find this. It would then be best not to repeat this routine.

11. If you do not experience any discomfort from performing this routine, then it would be advised that you perform it once a week for best result, but note that exfoliation on too regular a basis can cause skin irritation, so sticking to once a week is best.

Epsom Salt for Dislodging Blackheads

Blackheads are essentially a blockage of the skin's pores which can be caused by a number of everyday factors such as wearing makeup, sweating, environmental pollutants and incorrect or inadequate cleansing of the skin. The thing is that we all have them and due to the factors that cause them, it is very difficult to completely prevent getting blackheads, but it is definitely possible to remove them and keep them under wraps. Many commercial beauty routines that are designed to dislodge and remove blackheads can be very harsh and evasive to the skin, not to mention that many of them contain chemical additives that can cause irritation and sensitivity to the skin. The combination of Epsom salt and iodine provides you with a natural and non-evasive way of dislodging blackheads, resulting in a clear and glowing skin surface. To use this combination, do the following:

1. Dampen the skin on your face
2. Using ¼ Cup (60ml) Epsom salt, exfoliate your skin by gently rubbing the Epsom salt over your skin, this will remove any excess dirt and oil from your skin and prepare it for the treatment to follow
3. Rinse your skin thoroughly, taking care to remove all the excess Epsom salt

4. Take ½ Cup (125ml) of warm water (make sure it's not too hot) and dissolve 1 teaspoon (5ml) of Epsom salt into the warm water

5. Add four drops of iodine into the Epsom salt/warm water mixture and stir thoroughly

6. Massage the mixture into the skin, making sure you focus on the parts that are effected with blackheads

7. Allow your skin to naturally dry completely without rinsing off the Epsom salt/iodine solution

8. Once your skin has dried completely, rinse off the Epsom salt/iodine solution making sure that you have removed all the solution

9. Wash your skin as per your usual routine

10. Pat your skin dry and moisturize as normal

11. Depending on how bad your blackheads are you can perform this routine at least once a week, but it would not be recommended that you do it too often as it could cause your skin to dry out.

Epsom Salt as a natural face cleanser

Any effective beauty routine is not complete without a facial cleanser. As in most cases, many of the commercially available facial cleansing products contain fragrances and chemical additives, as well as preservatives that can be harmful and irritating to the skin, especially if you suffer from sensitive skin. Furthermore, many of the fragrances and chemical additives found in commercial products tend to have negative effects on the skin such as drying it out and in many cases can cause eczema.

Therefore, a natural face cleanser will always be your number one choice and is easier to achieve, and a lot more affordable, than one would generally think. Epsom salt provides a gentle and simple way of creating your very own facial cleanser which is best used as part of your normal nightly beauty routine and is done in the following way:

1. After you have performed your normal facial cleansing routine in your nighttime bath or shower, take 1 tablespoon (15ml) of warm water and place it into a cup or glass
2. Dissolve ½ teaspoon (2.5ml) of Epsom salt into the warm water

3. Dip a cotton wool pad into the Epsom salt solution and wipe it over your face in the same way as you would when applying your facial toner

4. Allow your skin to dry naturally before continuing with your moisturizing routine

Epsom Salt for Removing Styling Product Build up

For most of us a big part of our morning routine is styling our hair using products that are designed to hold our style in place. These are usually products such as hair spray, volume creating mousses, hair gels, and heat protecting products.

Unfortunately, by using these products on a daily basis they begin to build up in our hair to the point where our everyday shampoo is just not coping at doing the job of cleansing all these products out completely on its own. There is also the factor of chemical build-up from these commercial products to take into account, therefore it is indeed necessary to regularly perform a routine to cleanse the hair and remove all the buildup of these products.

The following routine will show you how Epsom salt, combined with lemon juice will provide you with an affordable and non-evasive way of thoroughly cleansing your hair of all this product buildup that is in question. This routine is then followed by a moisturizing routine that will help nourish your hair naturally; giving it softness and strength helping you to take full care of your crowning glory.

To remove the styling product buildup:

1. Take 1 Cup (250ml) Epsom Salt and 1 cup (250ml) fresh organic lemon juice
2. Dissolve the Epsom salt and lemon juice in 1 Gallon (5litres) of water
3. Cover the solution and allow to sit for twenty-four hours
4. After allowing the solution to sit for the required twenty-four-hour period, pour the solution over your hair, taking care to make sure that all of your hair is covered with the solution
5. Leave the solution on your hair for 15 to 20 minutes
6. Shampoo your hair as usual, but don't condition
7. Once you have finished shampooing your hair, pat it dry with a towel and comb it out
8. Cover your hair from root to tip with extra virgin coconut oil
9. If you have long hair it will be helpful to braid your hair and then pin it up
10. Leave the coconut oil in your hair for twenty-four hours, allowing your now completely cleansed hair to absorb all the moisture from the coconut oil
11. After twenty-four hours, shampoo and condition your hair as normal. You may need to shampoo twice in order to remove all the coconut oil

Epsom Salts to add volume to hair

One of the things most of us with fine hair crave is a head of hair that is full of volume and healthy bounce. There are many styling products on the commercial market that promise to help us achieve this, and they do so effectively.

However, the drawback of these commercially available styling products is that they are high in chemical additives that can not only cause a buildup in our hair, but also potentially decrease the natural strength of our hair.

By combining Epsom salt with a sulfate-free conditioner (which is available at most retail stores, health stores, pharmacies, or salons) you can easily create healthy volume in your hair without using excessive amounts of styling products.

Here's how to do it:

1. Mix an equal part of Epsom salt with an equal part of all-natural sulfate-free hair conditioner
2. Warm the mixture by rubbing it in your hands

3. Apply it to your damp hair, (this is best done after shampooing) and work it through your hair from root to tip

4. Allow it to sit for about five minutes before thoroughly rinsing off your hair

5. Dry and style as usual, you should notice that your hair now has a natural shine, body and bounce to it.

Chapter Three: Epsom Salt for Home and Garden

Epsom salt also has many uses within the home and garden that provide you with an alternative to the commercial chemical-based cleaning products and insecticides. This chapter will give you some innovative uses for Epsom salt around you home and in your garden that will be both cost-effective and harmless to your children and pets, yet will still get the job done just as efficiently as any commercial product will.

Epsom Salt to clean Pots and Pans

Many commercial cleaning products can be very abrasive due to them containing chemicals such as ammonia and certain types of alcohol. While these chemicals are essentially harmful to us, unless physically ingested, they can cause damage to your cookware over time. By using Epsom salt to clean your cookware you are taking a natural, yet softer, form of abrasion to the dirt that is stuck to your cookware. The Epsom salt will help dissolve the caked-on dirt without causing scratches or removing the non-stick coating of your cookware. To use Epsom salt as a cleaning agent for your pots and pans do the following:

1. Fill your kitchen sink with hot water, but not too hot that you can't put your hands in it
2. Add ½ cup (125ml) of Epsom salt to your dishwashing water
3. Place your cookware in the water and allow to soak for approximately 20 minutes
4. Wash your cookware in the Epsom salt water as usual, and rinse

Epsom Salt to Clean Tiles and Grouting

One of the most frustrating things about home maintenance is managing to keep bathroom tiles scum free and the grouting in between them free of stains at the same time. Unfortunately, the buildup of detergents and personal hygiene products will essentially always create a layer of scum on your shower tiles and the extensive exposure to water will cause stains within the grouting.

By using Epsom salt to clean your tiles and grouting you will be effectively and efficiently cleaning off all the scum buildup while removing those stubborn stains that get into the porous texture of the grouting. To use Epsom salts for cleaning your bathroom do the following:

1. Depending on the size of the area you are cleaning, mix equal parts of Epsom salt and white spirit vinegar together
2. The Epsom salt will fizz in the vinegar; this is normal
3. Place the mixture into a spray bottle and generously spray the areas that you want to clean with the Epsom salt/vinegar mixture
4. Allow it to soak in for about 30 minutes before scrubbing as you normally would

5. If the stains are really stubborn you can leave this solution on the tiles and grout to soak in for up to eight hours. It also may take more than one cleaning with this solution before all the stains are completely removed.

Epsom Salt as a natural homemade hand wash

One of the biggest draw backs of commercially made hand washes is that, although they may cleanse your hands and fight off germs effectively, they can be rather abrasive leaving your skin dry and itchy. The heavy fragrances that some of these hand washes may contain can also cause irritation to sensitive skin. Our hands are one part of our body that are always exposed to the elements, and one could argue that they are used the most during the day, therefore our hands are consistently coming into contact with germs and the elements which is why a sufficient cleansing hand wash is so necessary.

The following recipe for homemade hand wash uses Epsom salts and baby oil to create a cleansing hand wash that will effectively rid your hands of dirt and germs while gently moisturizing them at the same time. To make this homemade hand wash do the following:

1. You can either choose to reuse existing hand wash pump bottles, which is kinder to the environment as you are essentially recycling them, or you can buy some ready-to-use bottles from your pharmacy or home ware store

2. Fill each bottle half way with fragrance free baby oil

3. Fill each bottle the rest of the way with Epsom salt

4. Mix well and place wherever needed for a gentle, moisturizing hand cleanser

5. This hand cleanser can also be kept in your handbag for those times you are using a public bathroom and there is an empty soap dispenser

Epsom Salt to remove detergent buildup

One of the most essential appliances in our homes is the washing machine, along with the refrigerator and oven; there are many households in which the washing machine is used on a daily basis, especially if you have a large family. Nevertheless, even if you don't use your washing machine every day, over time there is bound to be a buildup of detergent and fabric softener in the machine. To clean your washing machine and rid it of the detergent buildup in question while using Epsom salts do the following:

1. Fill the soap powder dispenser of your washing machine with Epsom salt
2. Fill the fabric softener dispenser of your washing machine with white spirit vinegar
3. Run the washing machine empty on its hottest cycle
4. Once the hot cycle is finished, run the washing machine again (also empty) on a cold cycle
5. Once the cold cycle is finished, open the washing machine door and the soap dispensing drawer and leave open for twenty-four hours so that all can dry completely

Epsom Salt in the Garden

Epsom salt has many uses within the garden including use as a fertilizer, green booster for your lawn and as chemical free pesticide. Magnesium sulfate is pH neutral and can only boost the health of your soil and therefore the health of your plants. It is actually impossible to use too much Epsom salt in your garden, it is safe and easy to apply as well as being easily absorbed and broken down by both the soil and the plants. Here are some great uses for Epsom salt in your garden:

a) Epsom Salt to improve seed germination

The high content of magnesium in the Epsom salt aids in seed germination, making this a great element to add to your soil while preparing it for planting your seedlings, as it will boost the growing strength of the plant cell walls as your seedlings move through their germination process. To use Epsom salt while preparing your soil for planting do the following:

1. Use 1 Cup (250ml) of Epsom salt per 100 square feet of soil
2. Mix the salt into the soil while tilling it in preparation for planting your seedlings

b) Epsom salt to increase nutrient absorption

Something that is interesting about many of the commercially made up fertilizers is that they add magnesium to the mix in order to help the plants absorb nutrients from the soil, just as magnesium helps us absorb nutrients from our food sources. When taking the completely organic approach to your garden the use of Epsom salt in place of these commercially made up fertilizers is a great alternative. To use Epsom salt in this way you would do the following:

1. Use 1 Cup (250ml) of Epsom salt per 100 square feet of soil
2. Mix the salt into the soil while tilling it in preparation for planting your seedlings

c) Epsom Salt to counter transplant shock

Unfortunately, one of the things that is hardest to avoid when gardening is the shock that our plants and seedlings undergo while being transplanted from either pot to bed or bed to pot. This transplant shock results in the plant or seedlings beginning to wilt once they have been placed in their new environment. To use Epsom salt as a means of countering this shock do the following:

1. Use 1 Cup (250ml) of Epsom salt per 100 square feet of soil
2. Mix the salt into the soil while tilling it in preparation for planting your seedlings
3. It will also help to regularly feed your transplanted plants with about 1 teaspoon (5ml) of Epsom salt on a weekly basis until they have settled in their new environment

d) Epsom Salt for greener foliage

Just as the human body can show signs of nutrient deficiencies, so too can plants, when the leaves of plant begin to turn yellow, this is usually a sign that the plant has a magnesium deficiency since magnesium is essential for the production of chlorophyll, which is what makes a plant green. One of the best remedies for this is Epsom salt in the following way:

1. Measure the height of your plant
2. Sprinkle 1 Tablespoon (15ml) per 12 inches (30cm) of plant height around the base of the plant

3. Do this once a month until the plant has fully recovered and is in its greenest glory

e) Epsom Salt to prevent leaf curling

Leaf curling is another sign of a plant suffering from a magnesium deficiency and the high magnesium content of Epsom salt will help you remedy this in a natural and chemical-free way. To use Epsom salts to prevent and treat leaf curling do the following:

1. Mix two tablespoons (30ml) of Epsom salt with one gallon (5litres) of water
2. Place the Epsom salt solution in a spray bottle and spray directly onto the leaves
3. This can be done once per month until the plant has fully recovered and the leaves are no longer curling

f) Epsom Salt for the prevention and deterring of garden pests

One of the common known repellents for garden snails and slugs is straight forward salt, or sodium chloride, which is useful since it dehydrates the slugs and the snails causing them to literally shrivel up and die. If you are going for an approach that is not so harsh, you can sprinkle Epsom salt around the base of your garden beds as it will not have the same effect as sodium chloride, but it will cause and irritation to the common garden pests that will effectively keep them away from your plants.

g) Epsom Salt for abundant harvests

When growing plants that produce fruit and vegetables, Epsom salt can be incredibly useful and beneficial to the process of crop yield. By applying Epsom salt to the leaves of fruit and nut trees you are boosting their magnesium absorption, which will in turn produce tastier and sweeter fruits. This is best done in the following way:

1. Mix two tablespoons (30ml) of Epsom salt with one gallon (5litres) of water
2. Place the Epsom salt solution in a spray bottle and spray directly onto the leaves
3. This can be done once per month

Tomato plants are known to have magnesium deficiencies and this is due to the fact that the plant size ratio to fruit yield is so unbalanced, and many commercially available tomato fertilizers are too high in calcium and not high enough in magnesium. Epsom salt will also be a great remedy for this and can be applied to the plant in the following way:

1. Mix two tablespoons (30ml) of Epsom salt with one gallon (5litres) of water
2. Place the Epsom salt solution in a spray bottle and spray directly onto the leaves
3. This can be done once per month

Pepper plants are another plant that has an unbalanced plant to fruit yield ratio, resulting in them being prone to magnesium deficiencies. Pepper plants can be treated for this with the use of Epsom salt in the following way:

1. Sprinkle 1 Tablespoon (15ml) around the base of your pepper plant once per week

h) Epsom Salt for beautiful Roses

Roses thrive in magnesium rich soil and therefore will only benefit greatly by the addition of Epsom salt, it is said that magnesium aids in the production of rose blossoms as well as the health and stability of the wood of the rose plant. For best results while using Epsom salt with your roses do the following:

1. Sprinkle 1 Cup (250ml) Epsom salt at the bottom of the hole you have dug to plant your rose bush in
2. Plant your rose bush and fill the hole with soil
3. Sprinkle 1 Cup (250ml) Epsom salt around the base of the rose bush and water
4. Repeat step 4 once per month

Chapter Four: Epsom Salt and Essential Oils

As mentioned in chapter one, the best way to reap all the health benefits of Epsom salt for your body is to soak in a warm to hot bath in which you have dissolved the Epsom salt into the water. The combination of Epsom salt and essential oils will boost the health benefits of both the Epsom salt and the essential oil, and when adding this combination to your bath or hand wash you then are reaping all the benefits of both of these incredible health-boosting ingredients.

Essential oils work mainly on our sensory organs, particularly that of smell. There are a number of therapeutic benefits to the particular fragrances of certain oils, and because these essential oils are natural fragrances and not chemically derived, they are not irritating to sensitive skin; also their oil base will moisturize your skin rather than dry it out as most chemically derived fragrances will do.

However, essential oils are not only beneficial due to their fragrances, many of them hold other health benefiting properties such as antibacterial, antifungal, anti-inflammatory, anti-rheumatic, antioxidant, calmative, hypersensitive, and diuretic properties, just to name a few.

This chapter is all about the combination of Epsom salt and essential oils and included recipes to make your own homemade bath salts, hand washes and moisturizers.

Epsom Salt and Orange Essential Oil Bath Salt

Orange essential oil has many health benefiting properties such as anti-inflammatory, anti-depressant, anti-spasmodic, it is a natural antiseptic, a carminative, can have a sedative-like effect, can be used as a diuretic, and a general health tonic. Orange essential oil is also known for its anti-ageing properties. With all these amazing benefits of orange essential oil, this bath salt mix will make a great addition to your nighttime bath.

Ingredients:

- 4 Cups (1litre) Epsom Salt
- 2 Tablespoons (30ml) Orange Essential Oil

Instructions:

1. Place the Epsom salt into a mixing bowl
2. Add the orange essential oil
3. Mix together well, so that all the Epsom salt crystal are well coated with the orange essential oil

4. Place the bath salt mixture into a glass Mason jar and use as desired.

5. It is recommended that you add at least 1 cup (250ml) to your bath at any one time

6. This Epsom salt/orange essential oil mix can also be used on damp skin as gentle exfoliate; to do so take a handful of the Epsom salt/orange essential oil mix and rub it over your damp skin, rinse well and then shower as usual.

Epsom Salt and Juniper Berry Essential Oil Bath Salts

Juniper berry essential oil is known for its health benefiting properties such as; it is an antiseptic, anti-rheumatic, antispasmodic, calmative, and a diuretic. With its anti-rheumatic properties juniper berry oil will be a great addition to Epsom salt to make a bath salt mixture that will help relieve aching, tired joints and muscles making this bath salt combination a great addition to your after-training soak.

Ingredients:

- 4 Cups (1litre) Epsom Salt
- 2 Tablespoons (30ml) Juniper berry essential oil

Instructions:

1. Place the Epsom salt into a mixing bowl
2. Add the juniper berry essential oil
3. Mix together well, so that all the Epsom salt crystal are well coated with the orange essential oil

4. Place the bath salt mixture into a glass Mason jar and use as desired.

5. It is recommended that you add at least 1 cup (250ml) to your bath at any one time

6. This Epsom salt/juniper berry essential oil mix can also be used on damp skin as gentle exfoliate; to do so take a handful of the Epsom salt/ juniper berry essential oil mix and rub it over your damp skin, rinse well and then shower as usual.

Epsom Salt and Melissa Essential Oil Hand and Body Wash:

Melissa essential oil is known for its health benefiting properties such as; it is an antidepressant, has sedative-like properties, is a calmative and has hyposensitive properties. With all the benefits of Epsom salt, the addition of this essential oil is a great addition to your homemade hand and body wash.

Ingredients:

- 2 Cups (500ml) Pure baby oil
- 2 Cups (500ml) Epsom salt
- ¼ Cup (60ml) Melissa essential oil

Instructions:

1. Using a recycled shampoo or shower gel squeeze bottle that will hold a 2 cup (500ml) liquid capacity
2. Pour the pure baby oil into the squeeze bottle
3. Add the Epsom Salt
4. Add the Melissa Essential Oil

5. Shake well to ensure that all the ingredients are well mixed

6. Use as desired in place of your regular hand and body wash

Epsom Salt and Lavender Essential Oil Hand and Body Wash

Lavender essential oil is known for its health benefiting properties such as its ability to relieve and eliminate nervous tension, relieve pain, disinfect the skin and enhance respiratory function. Together with all the benefits of Epsom salt, this essential oil makes this homemade hand and body wash a very useful and beneficial combination.

Ingredients:

- 2 Cups (500ml) Pure baby oil
- 2 Cups (500ml) Epsom salt
- ¼ Cup (60ml) Lavender essential oil

Instructions:

1. Using a recycled shampoo or shower gel squeeze bottle that will hold a 2 cup (500ml) liquid capacity
2. Pour the pure baby oil into the squeeze bottle
3. Add the Epsom Salt

4. Add the Lavender Essential Oil

5. Shake well to ensure that all the ingredients are well mixed

6. Use as desired in place of your regular hand and body wash

Epsom Salt and Sage Essential Oil Hand and Body Wash

Sage essential oil is known for its health benefiting properties such as; it is an antifungal, antimicrobial, anti-oxidant, antiseptic, antibacterial and anti-inflammatory. Together with all the benefits of Epsom salt, sage essential oil makes for a great addition to any homemade hand and body wash, particularly due to its natural cleansing properties that won't be harsh and irritating to the skin. This is a very useful hand and body wash for active and sportspeople as it will help ensure that you are cleansing your skin of any bacteria that is caused by sweating, without stripping the skin of its natural oils or being too abrasive.

Ingredients:

- 2 Cups (500ml) Pure baby oil
- 2 Cups (500ml) Epsom salt
- ¼ Cup (60ml) Sage essential oil

Instructions:

1. Using a recycled shampoo or shower gel squeeze bottle that will hold a 2 cup (500ml) liquid capacity
2. Pour the pure baby oil into the squeeze bottle
3. Add the Epsom Salt
4. Add the Sage Essential Oil
5. Shake well to ensure that all the ingredients are well mixed
6. Use as desired in place of your regular hand and body wash

Epsom Salt and Orange Essential Oil Moisturizer

Because of the already mentioned anti-aging properties orange essential oil makes a great addition to any homemade moisturizer. One of the most important benefits of making your own moisturizer is that you are controlling what ingredients are used and therefore can make sure that it will not be harmful and irritating to your skin. This recipe uses pure aqueous cream as a base, which is free of perfume, paraffin, and any of the other chemical additives that many standard moisturizing creams contain; the addition of Epsom salt and orange essential oil to the mix make it a very beneficial combination to the overall health of your skin.

Ingredients:

- 2 cups (500ml) Pure aqueous cream
- 2 Cups (500ml) Epsom Salt
- ¼ Cup (60ml) Orange Essential Oil

Instructions:

1. Using a glass jar or a recycled aqueous cream tub, place the aqueous cream into the jar or tub

2. Add the Epsom salt

3. Add the orange essential oil

4. Mix together well

5. Use as desired on hands and body

Epsom Salt and Eucalyptus Essential Oil Moisturizer

Eucalyptus essential oil is known for its health benefits that include; anti-inflammatory, antispasmodic, antiseptic, and antibacterial. When combined with the high magnesium content of the Epsom salt, eucalyptus essential oil makes a great addition to any moisturizer or body care product that will be used by active people and sportspeople. This moisturizer also uses pure aqueous cream as a base, so it won't cause any irritation to sensitive skin.

Ingredients:

- 2 cups (500ml) Pure aqueous cream
- 2 Cups (500ml) Epsom Salt
- ¼ Cup (60ml) Eucalyptus Essential Oil

Instructions:

1. Using a glass jar or a recycled aqueous cream tub, place the aqueous cream into the jar or tub
2. Add the Epsom salt

3. Add the eucalyptus essential oil

4. Mix together well

5. Use as desired on hands and body

Epsom Salt and Lemongrass Essential Oil Moisturizer

Lemongrass essential oil is known for its health benefiting properties such as; it is an analgesic, antidepressant, antimicrobial, antiseptic, astringent, antibacterial and antifungal. Lemongrass essential oil is also known as a calmative, diuretic, insect repellent and has deodorizing properties. With all these benefits, lemongrass essential oil makes a great ingredient for any homemade moisturizer, and together with all the benefits of the Epsom salt, this moisturizer is useful to all walks of life. With its natural cleansing and antibacterial, as well as its insect repelling properties, this homemade moisturizer will be great to use all over your body and perfect for keeping in your handbag so that you have some with you all the time.

Ingredients:

- 2 cups (500ml) Pure aqueous cream
- 2 Cups (500ml) Epsom Salt
- ¼ Cup (60ml) Lemongrass Essential Oil

Instructions:

1. Using a glass jar or a recycled aqueous cream tub, place the aqueous cream into the jar or tub

2. Add the Epsom salt

3. Add the lemongrass essential oil

4. Mix together well

5. Use as desired on hands and body

Before you go, I'd like to remind you that there is a free, complimentary eBook waiting for you. Download it today to treat yourself to healthy, <u>gluten-free desserts and snacks</u> so that you never feel deprived again!

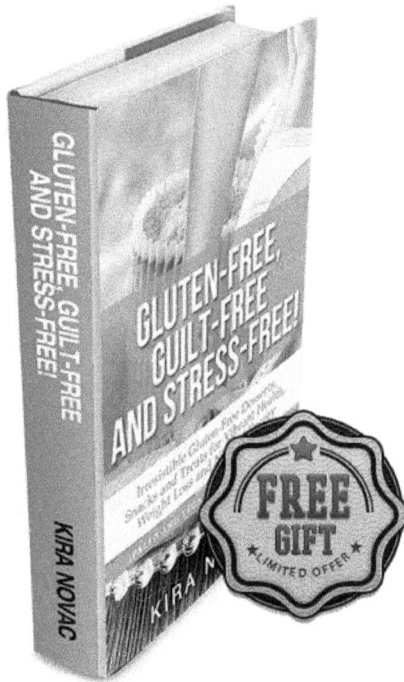

Download link

<u>http://bit.ly/gluten-free-desserts-book</u>

Conclusion

This book shows how this naturally occurring, incredibly affordable mineral, Epsom salt, is so useful and convenient to daily life in so many ways. We are constantly surrounded by gifts from Mother Nature and the modern world with its fast-paced commercial life has caused us to forget or become unaware of the natural compounds and elements around us that are so useful to us. The many uses of Epsom salt just proves how we don't have to only rely on commercially made chemical based products to live our everyday lives, run our households and take control of our health.

To post an honest review

One more thing... If you have received any value from this book, can you please rank it and post a short review? It only takes a few seconds really and it would really make my day. It's you I am writing for and your opinion is always much appreciated. In order to do so;

- Log into your account
- Search for my book on Amazon or check your orders/ or go to my author page at:

http://amazon.com/author/kira-novac

- Click on a book you have read, then click on "reviews" and "create your review".

I would love to hear from you!

If you happen to have any questions or doubts about this book, please e-mail me at:

kira.novac@kiraglutenfreerecipes.com

Recommended Reading

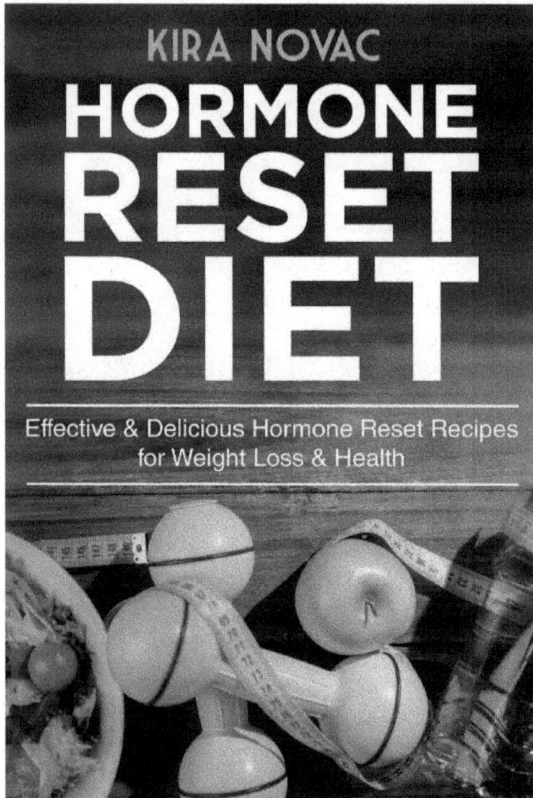

Book Link:

http://bit.ly/hormone-reset

Recommended Reading

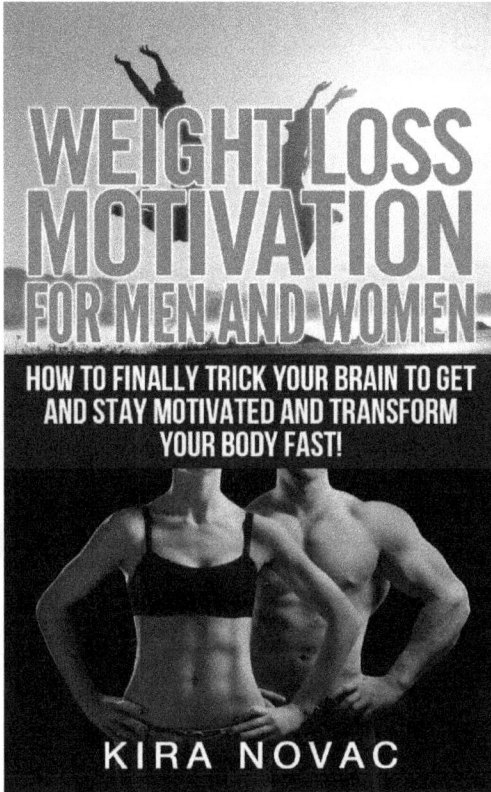

Book Link:

http://bit.ly/weight-loss-motivation-book

FOR MORE HEALTH BOOKS (KINDLE & PAPERBACK) BY KIRA NOVAC PLEASE VISIT:

www.kiraglutenfreerecipes.com/books

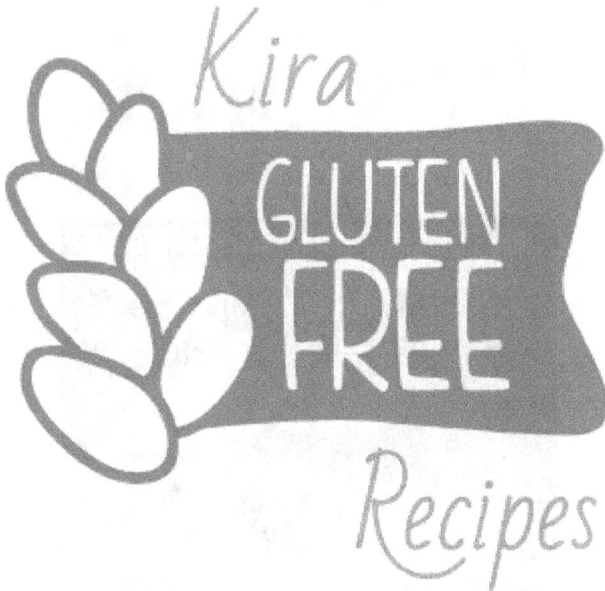

Thank you for taking an interest in my work,

Kira and Holistic Wellness Books

HOLISTIC WELLNESS & HEALTH BOOKS

If you are interested in health, wellness, spirituality and personal development, visit our page and be the first one to know about free and 0.99 eBooks:

www.HolisticWellnessBooks.com

www.ingramcontent.com/pod-product-compliance
Lightning Source LLC
Chambersburg PA
CBHW051039030426
42336CB00015B/2945